Hyper Ketosis for Beginners with Diabetes

A Balanced 21-Day Approach to Managing Blood Sugar, Weight, and Fatigue

mf

copyright © 2025 Mary Golanna

All rights reserved No part of this book may be reproduced, or stored in a retrieval system, or transmitted in any form or by any means, electronic, mechanical, photocopying, recording, or otherwise, without express written permission of the publisher.

Disclaimer

By reading this disclaimer, you are accepting the terms of the disclaimer in full. If you disagree with this disclaimer, please do not read the guide.

All of the content within this guide is provided for informational and educational purposes only, and should not be accepted as independent medical or other professional advice. The author is not a doctor, physician, nurse, mental health provider, or registered nutritionist/dietician. Therefore, using and reading this guide does not establish any form of a physician-patient relationship.

Always consult with a physician or another qualified health provider with any issues or questions you might have regarding any sort of medical condition. Do not ever disregard any qualified professional medical advice or delay seeking that advice because of anything you have read in this guide. The information in this guide is not intended to be any sort of medical advice and should not be used in lieu of any medical advice by a licensed and qualified medical professional.

The information in this guide has been compiled from a variety of known sources. However, the author cannot attest to or guarantee the accuracy of each source and thus should not be held liable for any errors or omissions.

You acknowledge that the publisher of this guide will not be held liable for any loss or damage of any kind incurred as a result of this guide or the reliance on any information provided within this guide. You acknowledge and agree that you assume all risk and responsibility for any action you undertake in response to the information in this guide.

Using this guide does not guarantee any particular result (e.g., weight loss or a cure). By reading this guide, you acknowledge that there are no guarantees to any specific outcome or results you can expect.

All product names, diet plans, or names used in this guide are for identification purposes only and are the property of their respective owners. The use of these names does not imply endorsement. All other trademarks cited herein are the property of their respective owners.

Where applicable, this guide is not intended to be a substitute for the original work of this diet plan and is, at most, a supplement to the original work for this diet plan and never a direct substitute. This guide is a personal expression of the facts of that diet plan.

Where applicable, persons shown in the cover images are stock photography models and the publisher has obtained the rights to use the images through license agreements with third-party stock image companies.

Table of Contents

Introduction   7
The Science Behind Hyper Ketosis and Diabetes   9
   What Is Hyper Ketosis, and Why Does It Matter for Diabetics? 9
   Nutritional Ketosis vs. Ketoacidosis   10
   How Ketosis Affects Blood Glucose and Insulin   11
   Why Low-Carb Works for Type 2 Diabetes   12
   Safety Concerns and Who Should NOT Try This   13
Getting Prepared – What You Need to Know Before Starting 16
   Speak with Your Doctor First   16
   What to Track: Blood Glucose, Ketones, and More   18
   Essential Tools for Success   21
Hyper Keto-Friendly Foods   24
   Low-Glycemic Vegetables and Proteins   24
   Fats That Support Energy and Brain Health   27
   The Best and Worst Sweeteners for Diabetics   28
Foods to Avoid and Why   31
   The Hidden Sugars That Spike Insulin   31
   Processed Keto Traps That Harm Diabetics   33
   Alcohol, Caffeine, and Other Triggers   35
The 21-Day Hyper Ketosis Plan (Diabetes-Safe Edition)   38
   Week 1 – Transitioning Into Ketosis Without Spiking Blood Sugar   38
   Week 2 – Fat-Adapting Phase   45
   Week 3 – Deep Ketosis and Maintenance   52
   Sample Grocery List and Meal Prep Tips   59
Sample Recipes for Diabetic-Friendly Hyper Ketosis   65
   Blood Sugar-Stabilizing Breakfasts   66
   Spinach and Cheese Omelette   66

Chia Seed Pudding	67
Avocado and Egg Bowl	68
Keto Green Smoothie	69
Fiber-Rich, Low-Impact Lunches	70
Zucchini Noodles with Pesto and Grilled Chicken	70
Cauliflower Rice Bowl	71
Keto Egg Salad Lettuce Wraps	72
Creamy Broccoli and Bacon Salad	73
High-Fat, Low-Carb Dinners	74
Salmon with Lemon Butter Sauce	74
Beef and Broccoli Stir Fry	75
Chicken Thighs with Cauliflower Mashed "Potatoes"	76
Eggplant Pizzas	77
Keto Treats Without the Glucose Spike	78
Dark Chocolate Almond Bark	78
Coconut Fat Bombs	79
Keto Cheesecake Bites	80
Peanut Butter Cookies	81
What to Expect (and How to Troubleshoot)	**82**
Common Side Effects and How to Fix Them	82
Adjusting Medication and Insulin Responsibly	85
How to Know You're in a Safe Ketosis Zone	86
Long-Term Lifestyle & Next Steps	**88**
When to Cycle Off Keto (and How to Reintroduce Carbs Safely)	88
Exercise Tips for Diabetics on Keto	90
Staying Motivated Without Obsessing Over Numbers	91
Conclusion	**93**
FAQs	**96**
References and Helpful Links	**99**

Introduction

Managing Type 2 diabetes comes with its own set of hurdles. Balancing blood sugar levels, managing weight, and battling constant fatigue can often feel overwhelming, like a problem with no clear solution. Beyond these physical demands, diabetes also affects emotional well-being and long-term health, leaving many wondering how to regain control.

Hyper Ketosis offers a practical, science-backed solution to common challenges. Instead of focusing on calorie counting or restrictive eating, it shifts how your body uses energy. By limiting carbs, your body burns fat as its main fuel, producing ketones. These ketones stabilize blood sugar, boost energy, and support long-term weight management. It's a method designed to create real metabolic improvements, especially for those with diabetes.

This guide is more than just a collection of information. It's a roadmap to help you start your Hyper Ketosis journey safely and effectively. You'll learn what you need to know before you begin, what foods to enjoy (and which to avoid), and how to implement diabetic-safe strategies. The step-by-step 21-day plan is tailored to simplify your transition, answering key questions and offering tools to troubleshoot potential challenges along the way.

In this guide, we will talk about the following:

- The Science Behind Hyper Ketosis and Diabetes
- Getting Prepared Before You Start
- Hyper Keto-Friendly Foods and Foods to Avoid
- A 21-Day Hyper Ketosis Plan for Diabetics
- Sample Recipes to Keep Meals Enjoyable
- Troubleshooting Common Issues
- Long-Term Lifestyle Tips & Next Steps

Managing diabetes is a personal, ongoing effort, but this guide aims to make it achievable for you. It offers clear guidance, practical tips, and a supportive framework to help you take control of your health. By the end of this guide, you'll feel prepared and confident to use Hyper Ketosis as part of your management plan. This is the beginning of a lasting, healthier approach to tackling Type 2 diabetes, one informed choice at a time.

The Science Behind Hyper Ketosis and Diabetes

Diabetes management hinges on regulating blood sugar levels and improving insulin function. Hyper Ketosis holds unique potential as a dietary strategy for achieving these objectives. This chapter dives into the science of Hyper Ketosis, what makes it effective for diabetes, and key safety precautions that allow you to approach this lifestyle with confidence.

What Is Hyper Ketosis, and Why Does It Matter for Diabetics?

Hyper Ketosis describes a metabolic state in which your body primarily uses *ketones* instead of glucose for energy. Ketones are molecules produced by the liver when you consume very few carbohydrates, burn fat for fuel, and limit glucose availability. This process may sound unfamiliar, but it's a natural response that supports energy needs when food intake shifts away from carbs.

For people with diabetes, particularly Type 2 diabetes, this state is impactful. Diabetes is marked by elevated blood sugar levels, stemming from insulin resistance (the body's reduced ability to respond to insulin) or insufficient insulin production. Hyperketosis addresses these problems by controlling glucose intake and using fat-derived energy instead. This leads to stabilized blood sugar, improved insulin sensitivity, and better overall metabolic health.

By following Hyper Ketosis, you can reduce the blood sugar fluctuations caused by carbohydrate consumption, helping both your pancreas and other systems work more efficiently. Over time, many individuals experience enhanced energy levels, reduced fatigue, and easier weight management.

Nutritional Ketosis vs. Ketoacidosis

Before embarking on any dietary approach, it is important to understand the difference between *nutritional ketosis* and *diabetic ketoacidosis (DKA)*. While they share similar terminology, they are very different states with vastly different implications for health.

- *Nutritional Ketosis* is the healthy state this guide focuses on. Blood ketone levels remain in a controlled range (usually between 0.5–3.0 mmol/L), glucose stays steady, and the body efficiently utilizes fat for fuel. This state promotes stable energy and is carefully managed through dietary adjustments.
- *Diabetic Ketoacidosis (DKA)*, by contrast, is a medical emergency. This occurs when ketones build up to

dangerously high levels (above 10 mmol/L), typically due to insufficient insulin in the body. DKA often results from conditions like untreated Type 1 diabetes or poor adherence to insulin therapy. It's accompanied by high blood sugar and symptoms such as dehydration, confusion, abdominal pain, or shortness of breath.

While DKA is dangerous, following a controlled Hyper Ketosis diet does not lead to this condition. Regular monitoring of blood glucose and ketones ensures you remain in the beneficial range of nutritional ketosis.

How Ketosis Affects Blood Glucose and Insulin

Hyper Ketosis can significantly influence how your body handles blood sugar and insulin. Here's how this shift works:

1. **Reducing Blood Sugar Levels**: By minimizing your intake of carbohydrates, the primary source of glucose is removed. Without a carb-heavy diet, the swings in blood sugar that occur after meals diminish. This creates a more stable glycemic profile, which can prevent complications associated with chronic hyperglycemia.
2. **Lowering Insulin Requirements**: When blood sugar levels are minimized, there's less need for insulin. Insulin facilitates the transport of glucose from the

bloodstream into cells for energy. However, when cells become resistant to insulin's effects (as in Type 2 diabetes), blood sugar remains elevated. Over time, a low-carb diet can help improve insulin sensitivity, reducing the body's demand for this hormone.

3. **Increasing Fat Utilization**: Once the liver begins producing ketones from stored fat, your body maintains energy without relying on glucose. This shift has additional benefits, such as promoting fat loss and reducing reliance on stored glycogen.

Ketosis helps stabilize blood sugar, reduce insulin needs, and promote fat utilization, making it a powerful metabolic shift. By minimizing carbs, the body improves insulin sensitivity and relies on fat for energy, offering potential benefits for overall health.

Why Low-Carb Works for Type 2 Diabetes

Although traditional dietary guidelines often promote "everything in moderation," research shows that reducing carbohydrates is one of the most effective ways to control Type 2 diabetes. Here's why:

1. **Carbs Raise Blood Sugar Most Rapidly**

   Carbs, especially refined and starchy ones, quickly break down into glucose, causing a spike in blood sugar. By limiting them, you avoid these sharp increases and the subsequent energy crashes.

2. **Reduces the Need for High Insulin Production**

   When you eat high-carb meals, your insulin levels must rise to regulate blood sugar. Over time, this overproduction can lead to insulin resistance. A low-carb diet minimizes this need, helping your body reset its insulin response.

3. **Encourages Fat Loss**

   Excess weight is a significant factor in diabetes progression. By adopting a low-carb approach, you not only reduce glucose levels but also stimulate fat burning. This can result in sustainable weight loss, which improves your overall insulin sensitivity.

Low-carb diets are particularly effective because they address the root cause of Type 2 diabetes rather than just managing its symptoms.

Safety Concerns and Who Should NOT Try This

While Hyper Ketosis has helped many people, it isn't for everyone, and certain individuals should approach this diet with extra caution or avoid it altogether:

1. *Those with Type 1 Diabetes*: Hyper Ketosis may pose risks for individuals with Type 1 diabetes, as maintaining the right ketone and insulin balance requires precision to avoid the potential for DKA.

2. ***Pregnant or Breastfeeding Individuals***: Pregnancy and breastfeeding require sufficient energy and nutrients to support both the individual and the baby. The restrictive nature of a ketogenic diet may not meet these heightened nutritional requirements.
3. ***People with Kidney Issues***: Low-carb diets must be balanced properly to avoid excessive protein intake, which can strain kidneys. Individuals with compromised kidney function should avoid diets that are likely to exacerbate their condition.
4. ***Individuals with a History of Eating Disorders***: Highly restrictive diets may trigger unhealthy behaviors or mental health challenges related to food.
5. ***Specific Medical Conditions***: Some individuals with conditions like pancreatitis, gastrointestinal disease, or gallbladder disorders may find a high-fat diet worsens symptoms. Always consult a healthcare professional before starting Hyper Ketosis to evaluate personal risk factors.

Hyper Ketosis brings hope for many managing diabetes, thanks to its ability to stabilize blood sugar, improve insulin sensitivity, and promote sustainable energy. By fueling the body through fats and ketones instead of glucose, this metabolic switch creates a pathway for better health outcomes. However, as with any significant dietary change, understanding the science, acknowledging safety considerations, and working with a healthcare provider are essential steps to adopting this lifestyle safely and effectively.

Getting Prepared – What You Need to Know Before Starting

Starting any new lifestyle or dietary approach requires preparation, and this is especially important when managing diabetes. Hyper Ketosis can make a significant impact on blood sugar levels, energy, and overall health, but going in unprepared can lead to unnecessary challenges.

This chapter provides the foundational steps to ensure a smooth transition into a hyperketosis lifestyle. By consulting with your doctor, understanding what to monitor, and gathering the right tools, you'll be setting yourself up for success.

Speak with Your Doctor First

Your doctor is a critical partner in your health, and their guidance is essential when making dietary changes like Hyper Ketosis. Diabetes management involves multiple factors, including medication dosages, blood sugar readings, and overall health considerations. Because a low-carb, high-fat diet impacts these variables, medical supervision ensures that any adjustments are made safely and effectively.

Why Consultation Matters:

1. *Medication Adjustments*: If you're on medications such as insulin or oral hypoglycemic drugs, your dosages may need to be revised as your diet reduces blood sugar levels. Hyper Ketosis often lowers blood glucose significantly, so sticking to your current medication plan may risk hypoglycemia (low blood sugar). Your doctor can guide you in gradually tapering medications, if appropriate.
2. *Personalized Advice*: Medical recommendations vary according to your individual health profile. For example, if you have coexisting conditions such as high cholesterol, kidney concerns, or previous episodes of ketoacidosis, a doctor can assess whether Hyper Ketosis is a safe option for you.
3. *Close Monitoring*: Transitioning to Hyper Ketosis can lead to initial changes in how your body feels and functions, such as shifts in blood sugar levels, energy fluctuations, or electrolyte imbalances. By keeping your healthcare provider in the loop, these transitions can be managed with oversight and confidence.

Preparing for Your Appointment:
- Share your intentions to begin a Hyper Ketosis diet and explain your goals (e.g., improved blood sugar control or weight loss).
- Bring a record of your recent blood sugar readings, medication list, and any history of diabetes-related complications.
- Discuss potential side effects, such as the temporary "keto flu" or changes in electrolyte balance, so you know what to expect.

Working with your doctor provides peace of mind and a safer path forward as you begin this dietary lifestyle.

What to Track: Blood Glucose, Ketones, and More

Tracking progress is an integral part of successfully managing diabetes alongside Hyper Ketosis. By monitoring specific metrics, you'll gain insight into how your body is responding to dietary changes and can adjust your approach accordingly. Here's what to track and why it matters:

1. **Blood Glucose Levels**

    Blood glucose is perhaps the single most important metric for diabetics to monitor, as it provides a clear measure of how effectively you're maintaining stable blood sugar levels.

- ***When to Measure***: Check fasting blood glucose (in the morning before eating), 1–2 hours after meals (postprandial levels), and if you feel symptoms of hypo- or hyperglycemia.
- ***Ideal Range***: While targets vary by individual, fasting levels are often recommended between ***80–130 mg/dL***. Post-meal levels should ideally remain below ***180 mg/dL***.

Tracking your blood glucose helps you identify trends, such as whether certain meals cause spikes or dips, and it allows for quick adjustments to your diet or medications.

2. **Ketone Levels**

Ketones play a central role in Hyper Ketosis, signaling that your body has shifted from burning glucose to burning fat. Monitoring your ketone levels ensures you're within the safe, effective range for nutritional ketosis.

- ***How to Measure***: Use a blood ketone meter for the most accurate readings. These devices use test strips to measure ketone levels from a small blood sample.
- ***Optimal Range***: For nutritional ketosis, aim for ketone levels between ***0.5–3.0 mmol/L***. Levels

higher than this may require further investigation or adjustments.

Monitoring ketones regularly helps ensure you're in ketosis while avoiding risks like high ketone levels or ketoacidosis.

3. Daily Energy and Well-Being

While not as quantifiable as glucose or ketones, paying attention to how you feel is equally important. Note changes in energy levels, mental clarity, mood, or fatigue. Together with the measurable data, these qualitative observations can guide dietary tweaks.

4. Other Metrics (Optional)

Beyond glucose and ketones, tracking additional metrics like weight, blood pressure, or cholesterol may provide a broader picture of how Hyper Ketosis affects your overall health. Discuss with your doctor which data points are most relevant for you.

By tracking blood glucose, ketones, and other key metrics, you can better understand how your body responds to dietary changes and manage your health more effectively. Combine this data with how you feel day-to-day to make informed adjustments and stay on track with your goals.

Essential Tools for Success

Having the right tools on hand can simplify your transition into Hyper Ketosis and make tracking more manageable.

1. **Blood Glucose and Ketone Meter**

   A dual-purpose meter that measures both blood glucose and ketone levels is highly recommended. This ensures you can monitor both metrics using a single device. Look for a meter that is user-friendly, reliable, and compatible with the appropriate test strips.

2. **Test Strips**

   Ensure you have sufficient supplies of test strips for both blood glucose and ketone testing. Maintaining an ample supply allows you to track regularly without interruption, especially during the early days when more frequent testing may be necessary.

3. **Electrolyte Supplements**

   During the initial stages of Hyper Ketosis, many people experience a temporary imbalance in electrolytes, commonly referred to as the "keto flu." Supplementing with magnesium, potassium, and sodium can mitigate symptoms such as fatigue, cramps, or dizziness.

- *Magnesium*: Key for preventing muscle cramps and promoting relaxation.
- *Potassium*: Helps maintain fluid balance and muscle function.
- *Sodium*: Supports nerve function and prevents symptoms like headaches or lightheadedness.

These electrolytes can be consumed through supplements or food sources like avocados, bone broth, or leafy greens.

4. **Food Scale and Carb-Tracking App**

   A food scale ensures portion accuracy, which is helpful when calculating total carbohydrates in meals. Pair this with a carb-tracking app or journal to monitor your daily macronutrient intake. Many apps allow you to set goals for carbs, proteins, and fats, making it easy to stay within your targets for Hyper Ketosis.

5. **Meal Prep Containers**

   Meal preparation is a practical way to stay consistent with your dietary goals, especially in a busy schedule. Invest in portioned containers to pack and store keto-friendly meals in advance.

Preparing for Hyper Ketosis involves more than just changing the foods on your plate. By speaking with your doctor, knowing what to monitor, and investing in the right tools, you're building the foundation for a smoother transition, better results, and long-term sustainability. Proactive preparation empowers you to confidently manage your diabetes while embracing the benefits of this lifestyle.

Hyper Keto-Friendly Foods

A successful transition into Hyper Ketosis hinges on eating the right foods. Choosing nutrient-rich, low-carb options ensures your body remains in ketosis while also providing essential vitamins and minerals to support overall health. The foods you select influence your blood sugar stability, energy levels, and long-term success with this lifestyle. This chapter highlights low-glycemic vegetables and proteins, brain-supporting fats, and the best sweeteners for diabetics.

Low-Glycemic Vegetables and Proteins

The foundation of any Hyper Ketosis meal plan is choosing foods that won't cause sharp increases in blood sugar or insulin levels. Low-glycemic vegetables and proteins are ideal because they are nutritious, versatile, and support stable glucose control.

1. **Low-Glycemic Vegetables**

   Non-starchy vegetables should make up a significant portion of your meals. They are low in carbohydrates, high in fiber, and packed with vitamins, minerals, and antioxidants. Fiber is especially beneficial for diabetics as it helps regulate blood sugar by slowing the absorption of glucose.

Here are some excellent low-glycemic vegetable choices:

- *Leafy Greens*: Spinach, kale, arugula, and romaine lettuce are extremely low in carbs and versatile for salads, sautés, or smoothies.
- *Cruciferous Vegetables*: Broccoli, cauliflower, Brussels sprouts, and cabbage are loaded with fiber, making them satisfying and nutrient-dense options.
- *Zucchini and Summer Squash*: Perfect for grilling or as a substitute for pasta (e.g., zucchini noodles).
- *Bell Peppers*: While slightly sweeter, bell peppers are low in carbs and high in vitamin C.
- *Mushrooms*: These offer an earthy flavor and are rich in beneficial compounds.
- *Avocado*: Technically a fruit, it's a keto superstar thanks to its fiber and healthy fats.

Crucially, you'll want to avoid starchy vegetables like potatoes, sweet potatoes, and corn as they can quickly spike blood sugar and kick you out of ketosis.

2. Best Proteins for Hyper Ketosis

Proteins are essential for maintaining muscle mass, supporting cell repair, and keeping you full. However, overconsuming protein can lead to an increase in glucose production through a process called gluconeogenesis. For this reason, aim for moderate protein intake.

Good protein choices include:

- ***Fatty Fish***: Salmon, mackerel, sardines, and tuna are not only rich in protein but also omega-3 fatty acids, which reduce inflammation and support heart health. This is especially important for diabetics.
- ***Poultry***: Chicken and turkey are lean protein sources. Opt for thighs instead of breast meat if you want extra fat to meet your keto macro goals.
- ***Eggs***: A versatile protein source, eggs can be incorporated into almost any meal.
- ***Beef and Pork***: Grass-fed options are preferred for their higher omega-3 content. Cuts like ribeye, ground beef, and pork belly work well in a keto diet.
- ***Tofu and Tempeh***: These plant-based proteins are good alternatives for vegetarians and vegans.

- *Organ Meats*: Liver, heart, and kidney are nutrient powerhouses that provide essential vitamins like B12.

Stay mindful of preparation methods. Grill, roast, or bake proteins rather than breading or frying them in processed oils.

Fats That Support Energy and Brain Health

Fats make up the majority of your calories in a Hyper Ketosis diet, and rightly so. They are the primary energy source in ketosis and play a critical role in brain health, heart health, and satiety. The key is to choose high-quality fats that nourish the body rather than processed or inflammatory options.

Healthy Fats to Focus On:

1. *Monounsaturated Fats*:
   - Found in foods like avocados, olive oil, and macadamia nuts, these fats are associated with improved heart health and reduced inflammation.
   - Extra virgin olive oil can be used for salad dressings or light sautéing, while avocado oil is excellent for high-heat cooking.
2. *Omega-3 Fatty Acids*: Found in fatty fish, chia seeds, flaxseeds, and walnuts, omega-3s promote brain health and help lower systemic inflammation. For an added boost, consider a fish oil supplement.

3. ***Saturated Fats***: Found in coconut oil, grass-fed butter, ghee, and animal fats, saturated fats provide a quick, stable energy source. Coconut oil, in particular, contains MCTs (medium-chain triglycerides), which are rapidly converted into ketones.
4. ***Polyunsaturated Fats (in moderation)***: Found in nuts and seeds like almonds, pumpkin seeds, and sunflower seeds, these fats are beneficial in small amounts. Just be cautious with overconsumption and avoid seed oils like canola, which may cause inflammation.

Fats to Avoid:

- ***Trans Fats***: Found in margarine, shortening, and many processed foods, trans fats raise bad cholesterol (LDL) and lower good cholesterol (HDL), increasing heart disease risk.
- ***Highly Processed Seed Oils***: Oils like soybean, canola, corn, and grapeseed are high in omega-6 fatty acids, which can promote inflammation if consumed excessively.

Balancing your fat intake from various sources is key to meeting your dietary needs while supporting overall health.

The Best and Worst Sweeteners for Diabetics

One aspect of transitioning to Hyper Ketosis that challenges many people is reducing sugar intake. Fortunately, several sweeteners provide sweetness without spiking blood sugar, making them safe choices for diabetics. However, not all sugar substitutes are created equal.

Best Sweeteners for Hyper Ketosis:

1. *Stevia*: Derived from the leaves of the stevia plant, this natural sweetener is calorie-free, carb-free, and doesn't impact blood sugar levels. Liquid or powdered forms are excellent for beverages or baked goods.
2. *Erythritol*: A sugar alcohol with about 70% of the sweetness of sugar, erythritol contains very few carbs and has no effect on blood sugar. It's a popular choice for keto baking and desserts.
3. *Monk Fruit*: Monk fruit extract is another natural, carb-free sweetener. Its concentrated sweetness means you only need a small amount.
4. *Allulose*: This low-calorie sweetener tastes very similar to sugar but doesn't raise blood sugar or insulin levels. It's especially good for caramelizing or baking.

Sweeteners to Avoid:

- *Sugar and High-Fructose Corn Syrup*: Unsurprisingly, these are off-limits as they significantly raise blood sugar and can derail ketosis.
- *Agave Syrup*: While marketed as a healthy alternative, it's high in fructose, which can worsen insulin resistance.

- *Artificial Sweeteners (e.g., aspartame, sucralose)*: While these are technically low-carb, they may disrupt gut health and blood sugar regulation in some people.

Tips for Using Sweeteners:
- Use sweeteners sparingly and only when needed. Over-reliance can lead to cravings and hinder the development of a palate for natural, unprocessed foods.
- Experiment to see which sweetener works best for your needs, as sweetness levels and aftertastes can vary.

The types of foods you eat while transitioning into Hyper Ketosis set the tone for your success. Incorporating low-glycemic vegetables, high-quality proteins, healthy fats, and appropriate sweeteners provides a solid foundation for stabilizing blood sugar and maintaining an enjoyable, sustainable diet. Armed with this knowledge, you're now ready to fill your kitchen and pantry with keto-friendly staples that fit your goals.

Foods to Avoid and Why

When it comes to maintaining Hyper Ketosis for diabetes management, choosing the right foods is as important as avoiding those that can disrupt your progress. Certain foods, drinks, and ingredients may look harmless but can have a significant negative impact on your blood sugar levels, insulin sensitivity, and overall health. This chapter identifies hidden sugars, harmful processed keto products, and other triggers like alcohol and caffeine so that you can make informed decisions for your health.

The Hidden Sugars That Spike Insulin

For anyone managing diabetes, hidden sugars are a major pitfall. These sugars are often found in foods marketed as "healthy" or even "low-carb," making them easy to overlook. The problem with hidden sugars is their ability to trigger spikes in blood sugar and insulin, which can knock you out of ketosis and lead to fatigue, cravings, and disrupted blood sugar balance.

Where Hidden Sugars Lurk

1. *Packaged Foods*: Salad dressings, ketchup, marinades, soups, and low-fat snacks often contain added sugars to enhance flavor. Check labels carefully for ingredients like "cane sugar," "corn syrup," "maltodextrin," "dextrose," and "honey."
2. *"Healthy" Snacks*: Granola bars, fruit yogurts, and dried fruits may appear healthy but are often loaded with sugars that raise blood glucose quickly.
3. *Beverages*: Many drinks, including flavored waters, fruit juices, sports drinks, and non-diet sodas, are sugar-laden. Even fruit smoothies can pack a surprising amount of sugar due to hidden sweeteners or high-carb fruits.
4. *Processed Meats*: Some cured meats, like bacon, sausage, and deli meats, are made with sugar in the curing process. Look for varieties specifically labeled as sugar-free or free of added sugar.

How to Avoid Them

- *Read Nutrition Labels*: Look for total carbohydrates and added sugar content. Aim for products with 2 grams of sugar or less per serving.
- *Watch for Alias Names*: Learn to recognize alternative names for sugar (e.g., agave nectar, molasses, rice syrup), which can disguise added sugars in ingredient lists.

- *Limit Packaged Foods*: Whenever possible, opt for whole, unprocessed foods like fresh vegetables, meats, and healthy fats.

Processed Keto Traps That Harm Diabetics

The popularity of the ketogenic diet has led to a surge in pre-packaged "keto-friendly" foods. While convenient, many of these products can undermine your goal of managing diabetes through Hyper Ketosis. They can sneak in ingredients that hinder ketosis, spike insulin, or harm digestion.

Common Processed Keto Pitfalls

1. *Keto Bars and Snacks*: Many keto snacks use sugar alcohols like maltitol, which can raise blood sugar in diabetics. Additionally, these products may contain artificial flavors, low-quality fats, or hidden carbohydrates.
2. *Protein Powders and Shakes*: Not all protein powders are created equal, and many contain added sugars, fillers, or high-carb protein sources like rice or pea protein.
3. *Nut and Seed Butters*: While nuts and seeds are keto-friendly, some products add sugar or hydrogenated oils, turning these healthy options into harmful ones.

4. ***Low-Carb Baked Goods***: Premade keto breads, cookies, and crackers often rely on starches or hidden sweeteners like tapioca flour or hidden syrups that can spike your blood sugar.

The Problem with Overprocessed Ingredients

Even if a product meets the macro requirements for ketosis (low carbohydrates, moderate protein, high fat), it can still harm your progress and health. Low-quality processed ingredients may:

- Trigger inflammation, which interferes with insulin sensitivity.
- Contain "empty calories" that fail to provide essential nutrients.
- Fuel cravings for sweets, making it harder to stick to the diet long-term.

How to Avoid These Traps

- ***Check Ingredient Lists***: Avoid products with maltitol, corn fiber, tapioca flour, or unhealthy oils like soybean or canola oil.
- ***Cook at Home***: Focus on homemade meals to have full control over what goes into your food.
- ***Prioritize Whole Foods***: Stick to single-ingredient items like fresh vegetables, raw nuts, high-quality meats, and healthy fats.

Alcohol, Caffeine, and Other Triggers

While these beverages may seem unrelated to your food choices, alcohol, caffeine, and other dietary triggers can directly affect ketosis, blood sugar stability, and overall well-being. Moderation and informed choices are key when incorporating these substances into a Hyper Ketosis lifestyle.

Alcohol

Alcohol can disrupt ketosis, interfere with blood sugar regulation, and impact weight loss goals. When consumed, alcohol is prioritized as a fuel source by the liver, temporarily halting fat burning and ketone production. Certain alcoholic beverages are worse than others for diabetics:

- *High-Sugar Options to Avoid*: Sweet wines, cocktails with mixers, flavored liqueurs, and regular beers are loaded with carbohydrates and sugars that can spike blood sugar.
- *Better Choices*: Dry wines, champagne, and hard liquors like vodka, gin, or whiskey contain little to no carbs. Just be sure to drink them straight or with sugar-free mixers like sparkling water.

Caffeine

Caffeine, commonly consumed in coffee or tea, can be a helpful stimulant but should be approached with caution by diabetics. Excessive caffeine intake can:

- Increase stress hormones like cortisol, which may raise blood sugar levels in some individuals.
- Interfere with sleep, which is vital for blood sugar control and energy levels.

Other Triggers

Certain "healthy" components may still pose issues for some diabetics:

- *Artificial Sweeteners*: While they don't raise blood sugar directly, sweeteners like aspartame or sucralose can disrupt gut health and insulin response in susceptible individuals.
- *High-Oxalate Foods*: Some keto-friendly foods, like spinach, almonds, and cacao, are high in oxalates. These can lead to kidney issues if consumed in excess.
- *High-Sodium Processed Foods*: While sodium is essential on keto, too much from processed foods like deli meats and canned soups can harm blood pressure levels for diabetics with hypertension.

How to Manage Triggers

- *Limit Alcohol and Prioritize Low-Carb Varieties*: If you plan to drink, stick to small amounts of dry wine or sugar-free spirits.
- *Practice Moderation with Caffeine*: Aim for 1–2 cups of coffee or tea per day, and monitor its effects on your blood sugar and sleep.

- ***Be Mindful of Additives***: Pay close attention to labels when using sweeteners or processed foods to minimize hidden risks.

Avoiding hidden sugars, processed keto traps, and dietary triggers like alcohol or excessive caffeine can help you maintain safer blood sugar levels, support ketosis, and promote well-being. Understanding these pitfalls prepares you for grocery shopping, meal planning, and dining out with confidence. By steering clear of unhelpful ingredients and prioritizing whole, nutrient-dense foods, you reduce unnecessary risks and maximize the benefits of Hyper Ketosis in managing your diabetes.

The 21-Day Hyper Ketosis Plan (Diabetes-Safe Edition)

This 21-day plan is designed to help you safely transition into Hyper Ketosis as part of your diabetes management routine. By gradually adjusting your lifestyle, you'll ease your body into ketosis, adapt to burning fat for fuel, and set up sustainable habits for long-term success. Each week builds upon the last, with daily steps to guide you through this process.

Week 1 – Transitioning Into Ketosis Without Spiking Blood Sugar

The first week of the Hyper Ketosis plan focuses on easing your body into using fats instead of carbs for energy. By gradually reducing carbs and adding healthy fats, you can avoid blood sugar swings and minimize symptoms like fatigue or "keto flu." This week includes meal suggestions, tips for a smooth transition, and advice on tracking your progress.

Day 1 - Start Small and Steady

Goals for Today

- Begin reducing your daily carb intake to 75–100g.
- Replace obvious sugar sources (sweets, sodas) with keto-friendly options.

Meal Plan

- **Breakfast**: Scrambled eggs with spinach cooked in olive oil, a side of half an avocado.
- **Snack**: A handful of raw almonds.
- **Lunch**: Grilled chicken breast with a large salad (add mixed greens, cucumbers, and olive oil dressing).
- **Dinner**: Baked salmon with steamed broccoli and a drizzle of melted butter.

Tips for Day 1

- Hydration is key. Drink at least 8–10 glasses of water to begin flushing out excess stored carbs and water weight.
- Test your blood sugar before and 2 hours after your largest meal to understand how food affects your glucose levels.
- Take notes on how you feel, especially your energy and focus.

Day 2 - Ditch Hidden Sugars

Goals for Today

- Eliminate hidden sugar sources such as flavored yogurt, granola, or sugary sauces.
- Incorporate more whole, unprocessed foods.

Meal Plan

- **Breakfast**: Chia seed pudding made with unsweetened almond milk, topped with a sprinkle of stevia and a few blueberries.
- **Snack**: 1 hard-boiled egg and a stick of celery with almond butter.
- **Lunch**: Turkey and lettuce wraps (use romaine as the wrap, fill with turkey slices, avocado, and mustard).
- **Dinner**: Seasoned ground beef stir-fried with zucchini noodles in coconut oil.

Tips for Day 2

- Read food labels carefully. Many "healthy" foods contain added sugars or hidden carbs.
- If you feel cravings, focus on fats like avocado slices or a spoonful of coconut oil instead of reaching for snacks.
- Continue tracking your blood sugar and write down how your meals impact energy levels.

Day 3 - Add Electrolytes and Monitor Progress
Goals for Today

- Maintain carb intake below 75g while incorporating essential electrolytes (sodium, potassium, magnesium).
- Start tracking ketone levels with simple urine test strips.

Meal Plan

- **Breakfast**: Two fried eggs with sautéed mushrooms and a side of bacon (unsweetened).
- **Snack**: 1 small handful of macadamia nuts.
- **Lunch**: Grilled salmon over spinach with olive oil, lemon, and sunflower seeds.
- **Dinner**: Cauliflower rice stir-fried in coconut oil with diced chicken and broccoli.

Tips for Day 3

- Add a pinch of salt or electrolyte drops to your water to prevent symptoms of the "keto flu."
- Experiment with tracking ketones for the first time today. Early stages may show low levels, but that's okay.

Day 4 - Stay Consistent
- Goals for Today
- Keep carbs consistent around 50–70g.

- Focus on meal prepping for the next 2–3 days to stay on track.

Meal Plan

- **Breakfast**: Omelet stuffed with spinach, bell peppers, and feta cheese, cooked in ghee.
- **Snack**: Celery sticks with cream cheese.
- **Lunch**: Grilled chicken thigh with roasted asparagus and a mixed greens salad.
- **Dinner**: Pork chops with mashed cauliflower and a side of sautéed kale.

Tips for Day 4

- Combat fatigue by eating magnesium-rich foods like leafy greens and almonds or take a magnesium supplement.
- If hunger between meals persists, increase your fat intake rather than snacking excessively.

Day 5 - Adjust and Fine-Tune

Goals for Today

- Reduce carbs slightly to around 50g, if you're ready.
- Identify foods that stabilize your blood sugar and make you feel energized.

Meal Plan

- **Breakfast**: Keto smoothie with unsweetened almond milk, ½ avocado, spinach, and a scoop of unsweetened protein powder.
- **Snack**: Keto fat bomb (made with coconut oil, cocoa powder, and a touch of stevia).
- **Lunch**: Pan-seared chicken thighs with roasted Brussels sprouts.
- **Dinner**: Grilled shrimp skewers with zucchini and cherry tomatoes, drizzled with olive oil.

Tips for Day 5

Pay close attention to how your body responds to the lower carb intake. If you feel weak or shaky, add 10–15g of carbs in the form of non-starchy vegetables.

Day 6 - Experiment With a 12-Hour Fast

Goals for Today

- Extend your overnight fasting window to 12 hours (e.g., finish dinner by 7 PM and delay breakfast until 7 AM).
- Continue reducing carb intake to 50g or below.

Meal Plan

- **Breakfast (after fasting)**: 2 boiled eggs, ½ avocado, and a handful of sautéed spinach.
- **Snack**: Olives or cheese cubes.

- **Lunch**: Turkey burger patty with a side of zucchini fries (baked, not fried).
- **Dinner**: Grilled salmon with a creamy cauliflower mash and roasted asparagus.

Tips for Day 6

- If fasting feels difficult, try drinking water or herbal tea to manage hunger in the morning.
- Monitor your blood sugar levels carefully today to ensure fasting doesn't cause dips.

Day 7 - Prep for Week 2

Goals for Today

- Reflect on Week 1 progress and how your body has responded to lower carb intake.
- Plan and prep meals for Week 2 to stay consistent.

Meal Plan

- *Breakfast*: Keto pancakes (made with almond flour) served with butter and a few raspberries.
- *Snack*: Handful of sunflower seeds.
- *Lunch*: Cobb salad (lettuce, boiled egg, avocado, grilled chicken, and olive oil dressing).
- *Dinner*: Beef stir-fry with colorful bell peppers and broccoli, cooked in coconut oil.

Tips for Day 7

- Review your ketone and blood sugar readings from the week. Are you seeing improvements in stability?
- Focus on meal prepping for Week 2. Cook proteins in bulk, chop vegetables, and make snacks like fat bombs for easy access.

By the end of Week 1, you should find it easier to stick to a low-carb lifestyle while keeping blood sugar levels stable. You might notice small shifts, such as fewer cravings, more stable energy, or slight improvements in weight and blood glucose readings. These small victories will help motivate you as you move into the Fat-Adapting Phase of Week 2.

Week 2 – Fat-Adapting Phase

Week 2 focuses on fat adaptation, where your body relies more on fat for energy, stabilizing blood sugar and supporting metabolic health. While challenges like cravings and low energy may arise, proper strategies and meal planning can help. Follow the day-by-day guide for tips, meals, and advice to deepen ketosis and manage diabetes effectively.

Day 8 - Lowering Carbs and Boosting Fats
Goals for Today

- Reduce net carbs to 40–50g.
- Focus on incorporating more healthy fats to keep you full and energized.

Meal Plan

- Breakfast: Two scrambled eggs with a side of sautéed kale and a slice of avocado.
- Snack: A handful of macadamia nuts or a boiled egg with a dash of salt.
- Lunch: Salad with grilled chicken, mixed greens, cucumbers, olive oil, and lemon juice.
- Dinner: Grilled salmon topped with garlic butter, served with roasted asparagus and a small side of cauliflower mash.

Tips for Day 8

- Avoid distractions like packaged "keto snacks," which can contain hidden carbs. Stick to whole, unprocessed fats and proteins.
- Track both blood sugar and ketones to see how your body responds to lower carbs.

Day 9 - Combatting Energy Dips

Goals for Today

- Continue at 40–50g of carbs.
- Focus on hydrating and replenishing electrolytes to prevent fatigue.

Meal Plan

- Breakfast: Chia seed pudding made with unsweetened coconut milk, topped with a sprinkle of cinnamon and a few raspberries.

- Snack: A celery stick filled with cream cheese or almond butter.
- Lunch: Turkey lettuce wraps with avocado and a side of sliced cucumbers.
- Dinner: Pan-seared chicken thighs with sautéed spinach and a drizzle of olive oil.

Tips for Day 9

If you start to feel light-headed or sluggish, it may be due to a loss of electrolytes (common as stored glycogen is depleted). Replenish with foods rich in potassium (e.g., spinach, avocado) or by drinking bone broth.

Day 10 - Managing Cravings

Goals for Today

- Prepare keto-friendly alternatives to your go-to comfort foods.
- Reduce carbs further (35–45g).

Meal Plan

- Breakfast: Keto smoothie with unsweetened almond milk, a scoop of protein powder, ½ avocado, and a handful of spinach.
- Snack: Fat bomb (made with coconut oil, cocoa powder, and monk fruit sweetener).
- Lunch: Grilled salmon salad with mixed greens, diced avocado, and a sprinkle of pumpkin seeds.

- Dinner: Zucchini noodles with a creamy Alfredo sauce (made from heavy cream and Parmesan), topped with grilled shrimp.

Tips for Day 10

- Cravings generally peak during this phase as your body adjusts. Use high-fat snacks, like a few slices of cheese or olives, to curb these cravings.
- Plan activities to avoid boredom-eating, like reading or taking a walk.

Day 11 - Testing Your Energy Limits

Goals for Today

- Experiment with a 12-hour fasting window to deepen ketosis.
- Stick to a consistent meal routine to stabilize energy.

Meal Plan

- Breakfast (after fasting window): Two fried eggs and a small serving of sautéed mushrooms in butter.
- Snack: A handful of Brazil nuts or a small slice of aged cheddar.
- Lunch: Grilled chicken drumsticks with steamed green beans, drizzled with ghee.
- Dinner: Pork tenderloin with roasted zucchini and a side of mashed cauliflower.

Tips for Day 11

If fasting leaves you feeling too hungry or fatigued, shorten the fasting window and eat a high-fat snack to sustain energy.

Day 12 - Paying Attention to Tracking

Goals for Today

- Monitor ketone levels more frequently to identify when you're in full ketosis (0.5–3.0 mmol/L is the goal).
- Fine-tune your carb and fat ratios to keep you satisfied.

Meal Plan

- Breakfast: An omelet stuffed with spinach, diced tomatoes, and feta, cooked in olive oil.
- Snack: Sliced cucumbers with guacamole.
- Lunch: Beef taco salad with ground beef (seasoned, no sugar added), lettuce, sour cream, and shredded cheese.
- Dinner: Grilled salmon with sautéed mushrooms and steamed broccoli, finished with garlic butter.

Tips for Day 12

Use a food-tracking app to ensure your macros are on point. Target 5–10% carbs, 15–25% protein, and 65–80% fat.

Day 13 - Overcoming Fatigue and Low Energy

Goals for Today

- Stay hydrated and include whole, unprocessed fats and proteins in meals.
- Prioritize sleep to allow your body to recover during this adaptation phase.

Meal Plan

- Breakfast: Keto pancakes made with almond flour, served with a pat of butter.
- Snack: A small handful of sunflower seeds or walnuts.
- Lunch: Tuna salad (made with avocado mayo) served in lettuce cups, with a side of cherry tomatoes.
- Dinner: Roast chicken thighs with roasted Brussels sprouts and a drizzle of tahini dressing.

Tips for Day 13

- If energy remains low, take a short walk. Light movement can boost both mood and blood circulation.
- Consider a magnesium supplement if muscle cramps or sleep disruptions occur.

Day 14 - Reflect and Prepare for Week 3

Goals for Today

- Lower carbs to 30–35g (if tolerable) to transition into a deeper state of ketosis.

- Take notes on how your body feels after two weeks on this plan.

Meal Plan

- Breakfast: Two scrambled eggs with diced avocado and a side of sautéed spinach.
- Snack: Pork rinds or cheese crisps for crunch!
- Lunch: Grass-fed beef patties wrapped in lettuce, served with a side of roasted cauliflower.
- Dinner: Cod fillets pan-fried in coconut oil, served with a side salad of mixed greens, cucumber, and olive oil dressing.

Tips for Day 14

By now, you should notice fewer cravings, more stable energy, and potential improvements in blood sugar levels. Reflect on your progress and celebrate how far you've come!

Week 2 is about perseverance and fine-tuning. As your body transitions into fat adaption, challenges like cravings and energy dips will gradually subside. You're preparing your body for deeper ketosis in Week 3, where you'll focus on maintenance and optional advanced techniques like intermittent fasting. Stay consistent, listen to your body, and keep tracking your progress!

Week 3 – Deep Ketosis and Maintenance

This week focuses on maintaining deep ketosis, exploring optional advanced strategies like extended fasting (if you're ready), and fine-tuning your plan for long-term success. The goal is to stabilize your blood sugar, maintain consistent energy, and build habits that will carry you beyond these three weeks.

Day 15 - Reducing Carbs Further

Goals for Today

- Lower carb intake to 20–30g daily (the ideal range for deep ketosis).
- Add more fats to ensure satiety throughout the day.

Meal Plan

- Breakfast: Two fried eggs cooked in butter, served with sautéed spinach and ¼ avocado.
- Snack: A handful of macadamia nuts or a small serving of olives.
- Lunch: Grilled chicken on a bed of mixed greens, topped with olive oil and a sprinkle of sunflower seeds.
- Dinner: Pan-seared salmon with creamy cauliflower mash and roasted zucchini.

Tips for Day 15

- Pay close attention to your satiety levels. If you feel hungry, it's okay to add an extra snack or increase the fat content in your meals.
- Keep monitoring your blood sugar and ketone levels to see the impact of deeper ketosis.

Day 16 - Testing Extended Fasting Windows

Goals for Today

- Try a 14–16 hour fasting window (e.g., finish dinner by 7 PM and delay breakfast until 9–11 AM).
- Focus on drinking plenty of water during your fasting period.

Meal Plan

- Breakfast (after fasting): Keto smoothie made with unsweetened almond milk, ½ avocado, spinach, and cocoa powder.
- Snack: Sliced cucumbers with guacamole or cream cheese.
- Lunch: Turkey patties wrapped in lettuce, served with a side of steamed broccoli drizzled with olive oil.
- Dinner: Roast pork loin with sautéed mushrooms and Brussels sprouts.

Tips for Day 16

- If you feel light-headed or overly hungry in the morning, break your fast earlier with a small high-fat snack like a boiled egg or a spoonful of almond butter.
- Slowly increase your fasting window over time if you're new to fasting. Don't push too hard; listen to your body.

Day 17 - Introducing New Recipes

Goals for Today

- Experiment with new keto-friendly recipes to keep meals exciting.
- Ensure you're getting fiber from non-starchy veggies to support digestion.

Meal Plan

- Breakfast: Keto waffles made with almond flour, topped with a small pat of butter and a few raspberries.
- Snack: A slice of cheese or a small handful of pumpkin seeds.
- Lunch: Zucchini lasagna (replace noodles with thinly sliced zucchini, layered with ground beef and cheese).
- Dinner: Cod baked with lemon and herbs, served with roasted cauliflower and asparagus.

Tips for Day 17

- Rotate your vegetables and proteins to keep nutrient variety; for example, try swapping chicken for turkey or asparagus for green beans.
- If digestion slows down, include more leafy greens and hydrate frequently.

Day 18 - Staying Consistent Without Overthinking

Goals for Today

- Stick to keto basics without obsessing over macros.
- Begin thinking about creating a sustainable plan for the future.

Meal Plan

- Breakfast: Egg muffin cups (whisk eggs with spinach, cheese, and sausage, then bake in a muffin tin).
- Snack: Beef jerky (ensure no added sugar in ingredients).
- Lunch: Cobb salad with chicken, boiled eggs, avocado, bacon, and olive oil dressing.
- Dinner: Grilled steak with roasted garlic cauliflower and roasted peppers.

Tips for Day 18

- Don't stress about hitting exact macro percentages. Focus on whole, unprocessed foods and ensuring you stay low-carb.

- Reflect on how your energy levels, cravings, and blood sugar control have changed.

Day 19 - Troubleshooting Plateaus

Goals for Today

- Identify any areas for improvement (e.g., sneaky hidden carbs or overeating keto-friendly snacks).
- Avoid over-snacking to ensure fat loss and blood sugar control.

Meal Plan

- Breakfast: Scrambled eggs with parsley and a side of sliced avocado.
- Snack: Two celery sticks filled with almond butter or cream cheese.
- Lunch: Tuna salad (made with avocado mayo), served on spinach leaves.
- Dinner: Baked chicken thighs with roasted Brussels sprouts and a drizzle of tahini sauce.

Tips for Day 19

- Use this day to troubleshoot any areas where progress feels stalled. Are you snacking too often? Are there hidden sugars in condiments? Adjust accordingly.
- If weight loss or blood sugar isn't consistently improving, reduce cheese, nuts, or fatty packaged foods and focus on basic whole foods.

Day 20 - Gearing Up for Long-Term Maintenance
Goals for Today

- Think about how you want to sustain this lifestyle beyond the 21-day plan.
- Refine portions and meal timing to suit your long-term goals.

Meal Plan

- Breakfast: Keto scrambled eggs with diced ham, sautéed bell peppers, and onions.
- Snack: A boiled egg or a few olives.
- Lunch: Grilled salmon with a side salad and a sprinkle of sunflower seeds.
- Dinner: Beef stir-fry with broccoli, zucchini, and coconut aminos.

Tips for Day 20

- Start making a list of meals, snacks, and strategies that worked best for you over the past three weeks.
- If you feel ready, test longer fasting windows (up to 18 hours) to see how your body responds.

Day 21 - Reflecting and Planning for the Future
Goals for Today

- Celebrate how far you've come in managing your diabetes and health.

- Create a realistic plan for either maintaining ketosis or cycling carbs (if needed).

Meal Plan

- **Breakfast**: Two fried eggs with sautéed Swiss chard and a side of sliced avocado.
- **Snack**: A handful of pecans or pumpkin seeds.
- **Lunch**: Grilled chicken Caesar salad (no croutons, with keto-friendly dressing).
- **Dinner**: Braised short ribs with roasted Brussels sprouts and cauliflower mash.

Tips for Day 21

- Reflect on what you've learned. Have your blood sugar levels stabilized? Has your energy improved? Take note of the positive changes.
- Celebrate your success! Even small wins are worth acknowledging, such as reduced cravings, stable glucose readings, or weight loss.

Week 3 is all about maintaining ketosis comfortably while setting yourself up for long-term sustainability. Whether you choose to remain in full ketosis or adopt a cyclical low-carb approach, the habits and knowledge you've gained can help you better manage your diabetes and overall health.

Sample Grocery List and Meal Prep Tips

If you're starting on the 21-day Hyper Ketosis plan, meal planning and strategic grocery shopping are essential to staying on track. The following grocery list ensures you have diabetes-safe, keto-friendly ingredients at hand, while the meal prep tips will make your week more manageable and stress-free.

Sample Grocery List

1. **Proteins**

   These are essential for maintaining lean muscle and satiety without spiking blood sugar.

   - Eggs (pasture-raised if possible)
   - Chicken thighs, drumsticks, or breasts (skin-on for extra fat)
   - Salmon (fresh or canned; wild-caught preferred)
   - Tuna (canned in olive oil)
   - Grass-fed ground beef or turkey
   - Pork chops or bacon (sugar-free and nitrate-free)
   - Sardines (packed in olive oil)
   - Deli meats (check for no added sugars or fillers)

2. **Low-Carb Vegetables**

   Focus on non-starchy, nutrient-dense veggies that are low in carbs and rich in fiber.

- Spinach
- Kale
- Swiss chard
- Broccoli
- Cauliflower
- Zucchini
- Asparagus
- Green beans
- Bell peppers
- Avocado
- Cucumber
- Mushrooms

3. **Fats and Oils**

Healthy fats are the backbone of a keto diet, and they'll be your body's primary energy source.

- Olive oil (extra virgin)
- Avocado oil
- Coconut oil
- Grass-fed butter or ghee
- Full-fat cream or unsweetened coconut milk
- Nut butters (almond or macadamia; ensure they're free of added sugars)
- MCT oil

4. **Snacks and Pantry Staples**

For quick snacks, cooking essentials, and flavor boosts.

- Raw nuts (almonds, macadamia, walnuts, pecans)
- Flaxseeds or chia seeds
- Coconut or almond flour
- Stevia or monk fruit sweetener (check carb content)
- Dark chocolate (85% cacao or higher)
- Bone broth
- Almond or coconut milk (unsweetened)
- Keto-friendly condiments (mustard, mayonnaise with no added sugar, vinegar)
- Pickles (fermented, no sugar added)

5. **Spices and Seasonings**

Seasonings help keep meals tasty without adding carbs.

- Sea salt or Himalayan pink salt
- Pepper (freshly ground)
- Garlic powder
- Paprika
- Curry powder
- Italian seasoning
- Chili flakes or cayenne
- Fresh herbs (parsley, basil, cilantro)

Meal Prep Tips

1. **Plan Your Meals Ahead**
    - Create a simple weekly menu. For example, plan 3 to 4 main recipes that you can rotate throughout the week.
    - Look for recipes with overlapping ingredients to save time and reduce waste. For example, prepare a batch of grilled chicken that you can use in salads, wraps (lettuce cups), or paired with sautéed vegetables.
2. **Batch Cook Proteins**
    - Roast or grill multiple servings of chicken, salmon, or beef patties at once. Store them in airtight containers for easy meal assembly.
    - Hard boil a dozen eggs at the start of the week. These make for quick grab-and-go breakfasts or mid-day snacks.
3. **Prep Vegetables in Advance**
    - Wash and chop your greens, zucchini, cauliflower, and other low-carb vegetables ahead of time. Store them in clear containers to easily assemble meals.
    - Consider roasting large trays of broccoli, cauliflower, and bell peppers with olive oil and seasoning. These can accompany any meal or serve as a filling side dish.

4. **Make Fat Bombs for Snacks**

   Fat bombs are handy to curb cravings and maintain your fat intake. Make a batch using a mix of coconut oil, cocoa powder, and a touch of stevia. Freeze them in silicone molds for portioned treats.

5. **Assemble Meal Kits**
   - Prepare single-serving containers with everything you need for a complete meal. For example, pack pre-cooked salmon, a handful of greens, and a small container of olive oil dressing in one container for a quick lunch.
   - Mason jar salads are another great option. Layer the dressing at the bottom, then add toppings like cooked chicken, cucumbers, and leafy greens at the top.

6. **Use a Slow Cooker or Instant Pot**

   These tools save time and make meal prep easier. Slow-cook beef stew or pork with keto-approved spices for a warm, ready-to-eat meal.

7. **Monitor Portions and Macros**

   Measure your fats carefully to ensure you're not over or under-consuming. For example, drizzle salads with exactly one tablespoon of olive oil or measure out a half-cup of broccoli for consistency.

8. **Have Keto Staples on Hand for Emergencies**

    Keep pantry snacks ready for when life gets busy (e.g., packs of nuts, canned fish, or jerky with no added sugar).

By shopping for these ingredients and following these prep strategies, you'll save time, reduce stress, and stay consistent with your 21-day plan while effectively managing your blood sugar and hitting your ketosis goals.

Sample Recipes for Diabetic-Friendly Hyper Ketosis

Here are some recipes tailored for Hyper Ketosis, divided into blood sugar-stabilizing breakfasts, fiber-rich low-impact lunches, high-fat low-carb dinners, and keto treats. Each recipe is simple, delicious, and crafted to maintain stable blood sugar levels while adhering to a keto-friendly diet.

Blood Sugar-Stabilizing Breakfasts

Spinach and Cheese Omelette

Ingredients:

- 3 large eggs
- 1 cup fresh spinach
- 1 tbsp olive oil or butter
- ¼ cup shredded cheddar cheese
- Pinch of salt and pepper

Instructions:

1. In a small mixing bowl, beat the eggs until well combined.
2. Heat olive oil or butter in a non-stick pan over medium heat.
3. Add the beaten eggs and tilt the pan to evenly distribute them.
4. Once the edges start to set, gently lift them with a spatula and let the uncooked egg run underneath.
5. When the omelette is almost set, add spinach on one half of it and fold the other half over it.
6. Sprinkle shredded cheddar cheese on top and cover the pan with a lid for 1-2 minutes until cheese melts.
7. Season with salt and pepper according to taste.
8. Serve hot.

Chia Seed Pudding

Ingredients:

- 2 tbsp chia seeds
- ½ cup unsweetened almond milk
- ½ tsp vanilla extract
- ½ tsp stevia or monk fruit sweetener
- Optional toppings: berries (small serving), unsweetened coconut flakes

Instructions:

1. In a bowl, mix chia seeds, almond milk, vanilla extract, and sweetener.
2. Let sit for 15 minutes to allow the chia seeds to absorb the liquid.
3. Stir well and top with optional toppings if desired.
4. Refrigerate for at least 2 hours or overnight before serving.

Avocado and Egg Bowl

Ingredients:

- 1 ripe avocado
- 2 boiled eggs, sliced
- 1 tbsp olive oil
- Sprinkle of salt, pepper, and paprika

Instructions:

1. Cut the avocado in half and remove the pit.
2. Scoop out some of the avocado to create a larger hole for the egg.
3. Place the sliced boiled eggs inside the holes of the avocado halves.
4. Drizzle with olive oil and sprinkle with salt, pepper, and paprika.
5. Bake at 375°F for 10-15 minutes until warmed through.
6. Serve as is or top with your favorite hot sauce for an extra kick.

Keto Green Smoothie

Ingredients:

- 1 cup spinach
- ½ cup unsweetened almond milk
- 2 tbsp unsweetened peanut butter or almond butter
- 1 tbsp MCT oil or coconut oil
- Ice cubes, optional

Instructions:

1. In a blender, add spinach, almond milk, nut butter, and MCT or coconut oil.
2. Blend until smooth and creamy.
3. Add ice cubes if desired for a chilled smoothie.
4. Pour into a glass and enjoy your keto-friendly green smoothie!

Fiber-Rich, Low-Impact Lunches

Zucchini Noodles with Pesto and Grilled Chicken

Ingredients:

- 1 medium zucchini, spiralized
- 1 grilled chicken breast, diced
- 2 tbsp keto-friendly pesto

Instructions:

1. Spiralize zucchini into noodles using a spiralizer.
2. Heat a pan over medium heat and add in the diced chicken breast, cooking until slightly browned.
3. Add in the zucchini noodles and cook for 2-3 minutes, stirring occasionally.
4. Once noodles are cooked, stir in pesto and cook for an additional minute.
5. Serve hot with salt and pepper to taste.

Cauliflower Rice Bowl

Ingredients:

- 1 cup cauliflower rice
- ½ cup sautéed bell peppers and onions
- 3 oz grilled shrimp
- 1 tbsp olive oil

Instructions:

1. In a pan, sauté cauliflower rice with olive oil until tender.
2. Add in bell peppers and onions and cook for an additional 3 minutes.
3. Top with grilled shrimp.

Keto Egg Salad Lettuce Wraps

Ingredients:

- 2 hard-boiled eggs, chopped
- 1 tbsp avocado mayo
- 1 tbsp Dijon mustard
- Romaine lettuce leaves

Instructions:

1. In a small bowl, mix together chopped eggs, mayo, and mustard.
2. Spoon mixture onto lettuce leaves and wrap tightly. Enjoy as a low-carb lunch option or snack!

Creamy Broccoli and Bacon Salad

Ingredients:

- 2 cups broccoli florets
- 2 slices cooked bacon, crumbled
- 2 tbsp full-fat sour cream
- 1 tbsp apple cider vinegar

Instructions:

1. Steam broccoli until tender. Mix with bacon, sour cream, and apple cider vinegar.
2. Serve as a side dish or add some protein like grilled chicken for a complete meal.

High-Fat, Low-Carb Dinners

Salmon with Lemon Butter Sauce

Ingredients:

- 1 salmon fillet
- 1 tbsp butter
- 1 tsp lemon juice

Instructions:

1. Season salmon with salt and pepper, then bake at 375°F for 15-20 minutes.
2. In a small saucepan, melt butter and add lemon juice.
3. Once salmon is cooked, pour lemon butter sauce over the top.
4. Serve with your choice of low-carb vegetables or a side salad.

Beef and Broccoli Stir Fry

Ingredients:

- 4 oz beef strips
- 1 cup broccoli florets
- 1 tbsp coconut oil
- 1 tbsp soy sauce or tamari

Instructions:

1. In a pan, heat coconut oil and add beef strips. Cook until browned.
2. Add broccoli florets and cook for 5 minutes.
3. Pour in soy sauce or tamari and stir to coat everything evenly.
4. Serve over cauliflower rice for a low-carb option.

Chicken Thighs with Cauliflower Mashed "Potatoes"

Ingredients:

- 2 chicken thighs
- 1 cup cauliflower, steamed
- 1 tbsp butter
- 1 tbsp heavy cream

Instructions:

1. Preheat oven to 375°F.
2. Season chicken thighs with desired spices and bake for 30 minutes.
3. In a separate pan, cook cauliflower until soft and mash with butter and heavy cream to create the "potatoes".
4. Serve chicken over the mashed cauliflower.

Eggplant Pizzas

Ingredients:

- 1 small eggplant, sliced
- 1 cup mozzarella cheese
- 3 tbsp sugar-free marinara sauce

Instructions:

1. Preheat oven to 375°F (190°C).
2. Place eggplant slices on a baking sheet and bake for 10 minutes.
3. Remove from oven and add marinara sauce and mozzarella cheese on top of each slice.
4. Bake for an additional 5–7 minutes, until cheese is melted.

Keto Treats Without the Glucose Spike

Dark Chocolate Almond Bark

Ingredients:

- ½ cup sugar-free dark chocolate
- ¼ cup almonds, chopped

Instructions:

1. Melt chocolate, mix with almonds, and spread on a baking sheet.
2. Refrigerate until hardened, then break into pieces.

Coconut Fat Bombs

Ingredients:

- ½ cup coconut oil
- ¼ cup unsweetened cocoa powder
- 1 tbsp stevia

Instructions:

1. Melt coconut oil in a saucepan.
2. Stir in cocoa powder and stevia until smooth.
3. Pour mixture into an ice cube tray or silicone mold.
4. Freeze for 30 minutes, then pop out of molds and store in the fridge.

Keto Cheesecake Bites

Ingredients:

- 4 oz cream cheese
- 1 tbsp stevia
- ½ tsp vanilla extract

Instructions:

1. Mix cream cheese, stevia, and vanilla extract.
2. Roll the mixture into small balls and freeze until firm.
3. Optional: coat in unsweetened cocoa powder or shredded coconut for added flavor and texture.

Peanut Butter Cookies

Ingredients:

- 1 cup unsweetened peanut butter
- 1 large egg
- 2 tbsp erythritol

Instructions:

1. Mix ingredients, form into balls, and flatten with a fork.
2. Bake at 350°F (175°C) for 10 minutes.

These recipes are designed to not only help stabilize blood sugar but also make your Hyper Ketosis lifestyle more enjoyable and achievable. Bon appétit!

What to Expect (and How to Troubleshoot)

Starting Hyper Ketosis is a big change for your body, especially when you're managing diabetes. While the benefits can be incredible, it's normal to experience some challenges or side effects along the way. This chapter will guide you through what to expect, how to handle issues that arise, and how to monitor your progress safely.

Common Side Effects and How to Fix Them

When you first start Hyper Ketosis, your body transitions from burning carbs for energy to using fat and ketones. This change can cause some temporary side effects, but most of them are manageable if you know what to do.

1. **The Keto Flu**

    The keto flu feels a lot like having a mild cold. You might notice fatigue, headaches, muscle cramps, or brain fog during the first week. This happens as your body adjusts to lower carbs and shifts energy sources.

How to Fix It:

- Stay hydrated. Drink plenty of water and add electrolytes (sodium, potassium, and magnesium) to your diet. Bone broth or electrolyte supplements can help.
- Eat enough healthy fats. Fat is your new fuel! Make sure you're eating avocados, nuts, and oils like olive or coconut.
- Get enough rest. Your energy might dip temporarily, so listen to your body and rest when you need to.

2. **Digestive Trouble**

You might experience changes like constipation or diarrhea when shifting to a high-fat, low-carb diet.

How to Fix It:

- Increase fiber intake. Eat more low-carb, fiber-rich veggies like broccoli, spinach, or zucchini. You can also try psyllium husk supplements.
- Stay hydrated. Drinking enough water is vital for digestion.
- Add probiotics. Foods like unsweetened yogurt, kefir, or kimchi can support gut health.

3. **Bad Breath (a.k.a. "Keto Breath")**

When your body makes ketones, one type called acetone can cause a fruity or metallic smell in your breath.

How to Fix It:

- Drink more water to flush out excess ketones.
- Chew sugar-free gum or mints made with keto-friendly sweeteners like xylitol.
- Don't worry too much–this usually goes away after a few weeks.

4. **Fatigue During Workouts**

Your energy levels may drop during intense exercise while your body adapts to keto.

How to Fix It:

- Eat a small keto-friendly snack before your workout, like a handful of nuts or a boiled egg.
- Be patient. Your endurance and energy will improve in a few weeks once your body adapts fully.

If any symptoms become severe or don't go away, contact your doctor to rule out other underlying issues.

Adjusting Medication and Insulin Responsibly

If you're taking medication or insulin for diabetes, starting Hyper Ketosis may change how your body needs support. Foods on this plan affect blood sugar differently, and over time, you may need less medication. However, adjusting these dosages is something you should NEVER do on your own.

What You Should Do:

- ***Work Closely with Your Doctor***: Before beginning Hyper Ketosis, talk with your healthcare provider about the potential need for medication adjustments. They can help you monitor your progress safely.
- ***Track Blood Sugar Regularly***: Check your blood sugar several times a day, especially in the early stages of ketosis. Share the results with your doctor so they can help adjust your treatment plan if needed.
- ***Avoid Sudden Changes***: Don't stop or change your medication without professional guidance. Even small adjustments can have a big impact on your blood sugar.

You may notice improvements in your blood sugar and insulin sensitivity within weeks of starting Hyper Ketosis. Stay in close communication with your healthcare provider to ensure safe and effective management.

How to Know You're in a Safe Ketosis Zone

When following Hyper Ketosis, you will want to ensure that you're maintaining a healthy level of ketones. This will help maximize benefits and avoid risks like ketoacidosis.

What Is the Safe Ketosis Zone?

- Nutritional ketosis for most people is a ketone range of 0.5–3.0 mmol/L in your blood (measured using a ketone meter).
- Ketoacidosis, on the other hand, happens when ketone levels climb dangerously high (above 10 mmol/L) and is usually accompanied by high blood sugar. This is rare for people with type 2 diabetes but requires immediate medical attention if it occurs.

Signs You're in Safe Ketosis

- Steady energy levels throughout the day.
- Controlled blood sugar levels within your target range.
- No signs of excessive thirst, dry skin, or confusion (these are signs of dehydration or ketoacidosis).

How to Measure Ketones

- Use a blood ketone meter for accurate results. Test once a day at the same time for consistency.
- You can also use urine ketone strips, but these are less reliable over time.

Tips to Stay in the Safe Zone

- Don't skip meals. Skipping meals can cause rapid drops or spikes in blood sugar.
- Stay hydrated and replenish electrolytes daily.
- Monitor both blood sugar and ketones together. This allows you to track how your body is responding and catch any issues early.

When to Seek Help

- If you experience extremely high blood sugar levels or ketones above 3.0 mmol/L, contact your doctor immediately.
- Symptoms like nausea, vomiting, or confusion may indicate a problem and should not be ignored.

Remember, the goal is to maintain consistency while keeping your body in a safe, healthy range. When managed correctly, Hyper Ketosis is a powerful tool to improve diabetes without compromising your safety.

With these troubleshooting tips and safety practices, you'll be well-prepared to handle the challenges that come with starting Hyper Ketosis. Most of the initial side effects are temporary, and your body will adjust as you stick with the plan. Stay patient, work with your doctor, and focus on your progress. You're on a path to better control and lasting health!

Long-Term Lifestyle & Next Steps

Hyper Ketosis is more than just a short-term diet; it can serve as a long-term tool for managing diabetes and overall health. This chapter explores sustainable ways to integrate keto into your lifestyle, adjust when necessary, and stay motivated without hyper-fixating on numbers.

When to Cycle Off Keto (and How to Reintroduce Carbs Safely)

While Hyper Ketosis can be a powerful tool for managing diabetes, it's not necessarily a permanent solution for everyone. There may come a time when you feel ready to adjust or cycle off the strict keto regimen. This could be due to personal goals, lifestyle changes, or simply wanting more flexibility in your diet.

The key to transitioning off keto is to do it slowly and thoughtfully to avoid blood sugar spikes or undoing the progress you've made. Here's how to reintroduce carbs safely and effectively:

1. ***Start Small and Choose Whole Foods***: Begin adding carbs back slowly, and focus on nutrient-rich, whole food sources like sweet potatoes, quinoa, or berries. Avoid processed or high-sugar foods, as these can cause sudden blood sugar spikes.
2. ***Increase Carbs Gradually***: Add about 10–20 grams of carbs per day for the first week and see how your body reacts. Keep tracking your blood sugar to ensure it remains stable. If all goes well, you can continue adding small amounts each week.
3. ***Pair Carbs with Protein or Fat***: To minimize blood sugar spikes, always pair your carbs with a healthy protein or fat source. For example, eat an apple with almond butter or quinoa with grilled chicken.
4. ***Monitor and Adjust Accordingly***: Pay attention to how your body feels and how your blood sugar responds. Adjust your carb intake as needed to maintain balance without overloading your system. Remember, this is not an all-or-nothing approach. You can reintroduce carbs while still maintaining elements of your keto lifestyle.

For some people, cycling on and off keto periodically may work best. For others, a "low-carb but not keto" approach might suit their long-term needs. The most important thing is to listen to your body and find what works for you.

Exercise Tips for Diabetics on Keto

Staying active is essential for managing diabetes, and exercise pairs wonderfully with a keto lifestyle. However, when your body relies on fat for fuel instead of glucose, your exercise habits may need some adjusting. Here are some tips to help you stay active safely and effectively:

1. ***Start with Low-Impact Activities***: If you're new to exercise or just starting keto, gentle activities like walking, yoga, or swimming are excellent options. These activities burn energy without putting too much strain on your body during the adjustment period.
2. ***Add Strength Training***: Building muscle helps improve insulin sensitivity and boosts your metabolism. Incorporate strength training exercises like bodyweight moves, free weights, or resistance bands 2–3 times a week.
3. ***Fuel Your Workouts Wisely***: While on keto, your energy might feel lower during high-intensity exercises like running or HIIT (high-intensity interval training), especially in the beginning. To prevent fatigue, eat a small keto-friendly snack before working out, such as a handful of nuts or a fat bomb.
4. ***Stay Hydrated and Replenish Electrolytes***: Keto can cause dehydration, so drink plenty of water before, during, and after exercise. Add electrolytes like

potassium and magnesium to prevent muscle cramps and exhaustion.
5. ***Experiment with Timing***: Some people find they have more energy for workouts in the morning, while others prefer exercising after a light keto meal. Experiment to see what feels best for you.

Always listen to your body. If you feel fatigued or dizzy, take a break and assess whether you need more calories, fats, or hydration. Over time, your body will adapt to using fat as its primary energy source, and you'll likely notice improved endurance and strength.

Staying Motivated Without Obsessing Over Numbers

Tracking your progress is important, but it's easy to get caught up in obsessing over numbers like weight, blood sugar, or ketone levels. This can lead to stress and burnout. Here's how to stay motivated while keeping things balanced:

1. ***Celebrate Non-Scale Victories***: Numbers don't tell the whole story. Focus on how you feel—more energy, better sleep, improved mood, or less reliance on medication. These wins matter as much as any metric.
2. ***Set Process Goals, Not Outcome Goals***: Skip the pressure of results like "I need to lose 10 pounds." Instead, set simple daily or weekly habits:
   - "I'll prep three low-carb meals this week."

- "I'll take a 20-minute walk every evening."

Focusing on actions gives you control and builds momentum.

3. ***Join a Community***: Support from others makes a huge difference. Find an online forum, a keto-friendly diabetes group, or a local walking club. Sharing progress and challenges keeps you motivated.
4. ***Be Kind to Yourself***: No one is perfect, and setbacks happen. If you have an off day or your progress slows, don't be hard on yourself. Learn from it and keep going. Progress isn't always a straight line.
5. ***Focus on the Bigger Picture***: Hyper Ketosis is a tool, not a perfect "cure." The goal is to manage diabetes sustainably while living a happy, balanced life. Remember why you started—to feel better, have more energy, and take control of your health.

With this guide, you have what you need to live a healthier, more empowered life. This is your journey—whether you stick with Hyper Ketosis, reintroduce carbs, or try new strategies, every step brings you closer to a stronger, healthier you.

Conclusion

Managing Type 2 diabetes is a challenging task, but you've taken an important step by exploring Hyper Ketosis as a tool for improving your health. This guide has armed you with the knowledge to better manage blood sugar levels, increase energy, and support sustainable weight management through this science-backed, low-carb lifestyle.

At its core, Hyper Ketosis is about shifting your body's fuel source from glucose to fat, creating a powerful metabolic change that can stabilize blood sugar and improve insulin sensitivity. Unlike crash diets or overly restrictive plans, this approach is designed to support your unique needs as someone managing diabetes. You've learned the fundamentals of ketosis, from what to eat and how to avoid pitfalls, to the science of how this lifestyle affects your blood glucose and insulin levels.

Preparation emerged as a key theme throughout the guide. From speaking with your doctor to gathering tools like a glucometer and electrolyte supplements, taking these steps ensures a smoother, safer transition. You've also seen how meal planning with keto-friendly foods can simplify your efforts, making it easier to stick to your goals while enjoying satisfying, nutritious meals.

You've been introduced to a practical 21-day plan and given tips for navigating potential challenges like fatigue, cravings, or digestive changes. These moments are a natural part of starting Hyper Ketosis, but as you've read, they're manageable with the right strategies. By properly adjusting medication, tracking metrics like blood glucose and ketones, and staying consistent, you can safely experience the benefits of ketosis.

However, this guide isn't just about the short-term. Building sustainable habits is crucial, and you now have the tools to adapt Hyper Ketosis to your lifestyle. Whether that means sticking with a strict ketogenic diet or cycling in carbs occasionally, the aim is to take control of your health in a way that works for you. Flexibility and balance, paired with mindful tracking and regular check-ins with your doctor, are your keys to long-term success.

Equally important is the mindset you bring to this lifestyle. Instead of chasing perfection, focus on consistency and celebrating small victories like stable blood sugar, better energy, or reduced cravings. Even minor improvements signify progress. And while individual results may vary, this guide has shown that acting with intention and staying informed can lead to meaningful changes.

Thank you for investing the time and energy to complete this guide. The effort you've put into learning and preparing shows your dedication to improving your health. Whether you're just starting or fine-tuning your approach, remember that this is your unique health journey, and you're in control of making empowered, informed choices.

The steps you take today can lead to profound improvements for tomorrow. Keep moving forward, stay curious, and don't hesitate to reach out for support when needed. Your health is a lifelong investment, and by implementing what you've learned, you're building a strong foundation for a healthier, more vibrant life.

FAQs

Is Hyper Ketosis safe for people with Type 2 diabetes?

Yes, Hyper Ketosis can be safe for many individuals with Type 2 diabetes when approached carefully. By reducing carb intake and emphasizing healthy fats, this method helps stabilize blood sugar and improve insulin sensitivity. However, since altering your diet can impact medications or insulin requirements, it's essential to consult with your doctor before starting to ensure safety and proper adjustments.

How do I start Hyper Ketosis?

To get started, gradually reduce your carb intake over a few days while increasing healthy fats, such as avocado, olive oil, and fatty fish. Ensure you're prepared with tools like a glucometer to monitor blood sugar, and consider tracking ketones with test strips or a blood ketone meter. Speak with your healthcare provider to create a diabetes-safe plan, and follow the 21-day step-by-step guide to ease into the lifestyle without drastic changes.

What foods should I eat on Hyper Ketosis?

Base your meals on low-carb, nutrient-dense foods. Focus on non-starchy vegetables (like spinach, broccoli, and zucchini), healthy fats (avocados, olive oil, butter), and high-quality proteins (salmon, chicken, eggs). Snack on nuts, seeds, or small portions of cheese. Avoid processed foods, added sugars, and starchy vegetables such as potatoes or corn.

What foods should I avoid, and why?

Steer clear of foods high in sugars and carbohydrates, such as bread, pasta, sugary drinks, and desserts. These can cause blood sugar spikes and kick you out of ketosis. Be cautious of "hidden carbs" in processed keto products or condiments like ketchup and marinades. Additionally, avoid harmful fats like trans fats or vegetable oils, as they can contribute to inflammation.

What side effects might I experience, and how can I manage them?

Common side effects during the initial phase of ketosis include fatigue, irritability, muscle cramps, and cravings (often referred to as the "keto flu"). These symptoms occur as your body transitions from burning carbs to burning fat. To manage side effects, hydrate often, replenish electrolytes with foods like avocados and spinach, and increase your fat intake to boost energy. Side effects are temporary and usually resolve within a week or two.

How do I track my progress and know I'm on the right path?

Track critical metrics like blood sugar levels and ketone levels to monitor your progress. Blood sugar should stabilize, while ketones should remain in the 0.5–3.0 mmol/L range. Pay attention to how you feel, too. Signs of success include improved energy, fewer blood sugar swings, reduced cravings, and gradual weight loss. Regularly check in with your healthcare provider for additional guidance.

Can I stay on Hyper Ketosis long-term, and what if I want to reintroduce carbs?

Yes, Hyper Ketosis can be a sustainable lifestyle for many, but it's essential to adapt it to your needs. If you wish to add carbs back in, do so slowly and in small amounts, starting with low-glycemic options like berries or sweet potatoes. Monitor your blood sugar and ketone levels to ensure you remain in control. Long-term success is about flexibility and finding a balance that works for you.

References and Helpful Links

Diabetic ketoacidosis - Symptoms & causes - Mayo Clinic. (2022, October 6). Mayo Clinic. https://www.mayoclinic.org/diseases-conditions/diabetic-ketoacidosis/symptoms-causes/syc-20371551

Fallabel, C. (2023, April 21). Understanding ketotic hyperglycemia. Healthline. https://www.healthline.com/health/ketotic-hyperglycemia

the Healthline Medical Network. (2024, February 29). A Guide to Healthy Low Carb Eating with Diabetes. Healthline. https://www.healthline.com/nutrition/low-carb-diet-for-diabetes

Ld, S. S. M. R. (2023, February 23). 20 foods to eat on the keto diet. Healthline. https://www.healthline.com/nutrition/ketogenic-diet-foods

Migala, J. (2024, November 27). 15 foods you can't eat on Keto (and what to choose instead). EverydayHealth.com. https://www.everydayhealth.com/ketogenic-diet/foods-you-can-t-eat-on-keto-and-what-to-choose-instead/

Ld, L. W. M. R. (2025b, January 24). 16 foods to avoid (or limit) on the keto diet. Healthline. https://www.healthline.com/nutrition/what-not-to-eat-on-keto

Hyper Ketosis Diet: A Complete Guide and Cookbook with . . .. (n.d.). Goodreads. https://www.goodreads.com/book/show/218412963-hyper-ketosis-diet

www.ingramcontent.com/pod-product-compliance
Lightning Source LLC
LaVergne TN
LVHW012030060526
838201LV00061B/4537